My Story
A Neuromuscular Disease and Its Human

John E. Tapper

2012 © John E. Tapper
Revised 2014
Sunburst Services, Houston, TX
Cover Art by MOZ ART & CO.

Printed by CreateSpace
ISBN: 978-1502935052
First Edition

All rights reserved
No part of this book may be reproduced
in any form without permission
in writing from the publisher, except in brief quotations.

*I dedicate this book to my wife
and partner of many years,
Idelle Tapper*

Dr. James Stringham, my mentor,

and

*those who battle with a variety
of neuromuscular diseases every day,
both at home and in the work place—
I call them fellow travelers—
they and their personal care workers.*

TABLE OF CONTENTS

A Long Journey With a Neuromuscular Disease....pg. 1

Assistance for Living

   Questions for Self Evaluation & Identifying New Options ...pg. 45

   Assistance for Living – Other Notes of Interest ... pg. 51

      Aquatic Therapy
      Service Opportunities
      Confronting Personal Stuff
      Equipping My Office

   Thoughts to Muse Over ... pg. 61
      Walls
      Frost
      Every One Has a Story
      An Elder's Statement
      A New Normal
      Peeling Paint
      Night
      Truggeling

My Story

A Neuromuscular Disease and Its Human

One summer, while sitting by the shore of a Minnesota lake watching the reflection of the northern lights dancing on the water, I became quite nostalgic and started to think about my life—past, present, and future. Later, while reminiscing about this event, my thoughts focused on **reviewing the employment side of my life and its relationship to my neuromuscular disease.** May what I have to share give the reader new insights into the world of physical disablement.

This Book was born out of my desire **to be a consultant to physically disabled people**. At this point I wish we could do some high-fives—only my hands don't work that way. I am like many of you—spending 16 hour days in an adjustable power wheelchair and 8 hour nights in a hospital bed. Of course, I had no choice in this matter. However, my body didn't always operate this way. Yes, I did **inherit the extreme version of a neuromuscular disease—Charcot-Marie-Tooth disease, Type-1A (CMT)**—but it did not make its full-blown power-wheelchair-user appearance until 22 years ago (the leg braces, surgery, canes, walkers and motorized scooters came first).

My name is John and I will share with you now an important part of my life's story. Please note that the "**bolding**" throughout this book is to draw your attention to significant changes in my employment—as they relate to physical changes taking place in my body. In other words, **my neuromuscular disease has been a powerful "decider" throughout my life.** Sometimes it was just lurking in the background and at other times taking center stage. My life has been characterized by the words "restrictions," "denial," "adjustment," "adaptability," "determination," and "thankfulness." I suspect that these words would also apply to many of you. **Life has been a constant physical struggle to compete on a daily basis.** At the end of "My Story" please take time to address the questions. **My intent is that they will stimulate you to develop personal workable options to consider when faced with Change-Points in your life.**

Many years ago I was born in cold country, Duluth, Minnesota, during the Great Depression. My heritage is Swedish/Northern European. Please note that the people of that era were **very stoic.** If times were hard, or you got hurt, just tough it out, ignore what you can, don't bother others with your problems and be thankful for what you do have. Contact with a doctor was extremely rare. Basically put, we were responsible for ourselves. But what about those times when one needed help beyond personal resources? Aside from family and maybe assistance from a church, synagogue or one of the few charities that existed, such help was a rarity. Smiles could become quite plastic. Things are different now, maybe—if you qualify.

Though I was busy during my childhood years, I noticed some differences between myself and childhood friends. I couldn't run as fast as they and I tripped a lot. In gym class I was repeatedly forced to try to do things that I could not physically do. For example, climbing a rope was out of the question but I was forced to try it to the point that I developed an intense dislike for gym. I had no advocate and was bullied a lot until I grew taller than most of my elementary school classmates. But, I could participate in several of the outdoor games that were popular in the '40's. By nature I enjoyed being active from dawn to dusk. I loved building model planes, etc. at my basement work bench. Our back yard was in terrible condition—housing a home-made wood fort complete with trap door—using scrap lumber. I dug out a fox hole and the fence was broken down. However, I did cut the grass using an old push mower. But basically speaking, my parents let me do my thing—with-in reason—physically speaking. SO-- ------------------------ I grew up with the idea that I could do anything that I set my mind to do – physically speaking. As you will discover through-out this book, such a mind-set can, at times, lead to unwise decision-making in the work place. I became an unrealistic optimist. In other words, the subtle irreversible loss of physical strength that I have experienced throughout my life – loss of strength caused by nerve degeneration – I found that I was not able to keep up with my dreams and goals. What I thought I would be able to do over a reasonable period of time – I soon discovered my body would not cooperate. It was a case of my mind running over my body. I trust that you will profit by these thoughts.

I need to insert an important statement at this point in time. I grew up in an era when medicine had limited understanding of neuro-muscular diseases. As a result, it was difficult for my parents to give good, long-range guidance to live by. They simply did the best they could with the knowledge they had.

At age 13, when I wanted to play football with my friends, the disease made its visible debut—**my right foot/ankle started turning over and my toes started to curl. Obviously, playing football with my friends didn't happen. At age 15 a double-bar steel leg brace for my right leg became part of my outfit. I was taught that the best way to handle my** physical situation was to ignore it—so I ignored it as best as I could.

My work life had a humble beginning. While in elementary school I went door-to-door throughout the neighborhood collecting garbage, then weeded out the returnable glass bottles which I brought to the neighborhood deli in exchange for a supply of penny candy. I don't think my mother appreciated the effort!

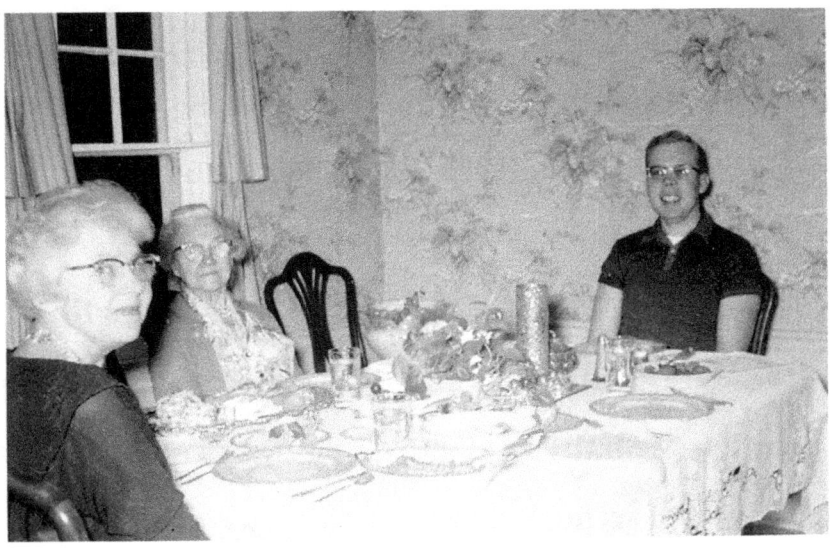

My mother, grandmother and me, in my late teens

Work that was approved, however, was in my early teens; **I delivered a local neighborhood newspaper** and did some **snow shoveling** in the winter—by this time we had lived in Minneapolis for several years. The year after high school was spent doing **heavy labor for my grandfather and uncle in their commercial laundry** which was located in a near north suburb of Chicago. It made no difference that I was living with a **painful, deformed right foot**. After gaining a little more wisdom, I decided to go to college—so this meant working in the laundry during the summers (but now I was old enough to **pick up and deliver** laundry, thus serving our customers when our regular drivers were on their summer vacations). During this period of time, and aside from that right foot problem, **I was quite strong—probably at the peak of my physical strength. I could force myself to climb up three flights of outside stairs carrying two heavy loads of finished laundry on my shoulder.**

My father passed away when I was a junior in college and I decided to delay taking the rest of my college courses. This meant spending several years working as a **tool-and-die-maker apprentice—in spite of my weak hands**. I was just following in the footsteps of two uncles who were highly skilled tool-and-die-makers. (I learned to compensate for my weak hands to the satisfaction of my boss.) Note that I worked under the close scrutiny of a tough old tobacco chewing Swede learning to make the dies, jigs, and fixtures that are used to manufacture products in a variety of industries. Of course, I also had to master learning how to operate the shop equipment. I was constantly having to prove myself physically capable to perform assigned duties. **The neuromuscular disease usually created a barrier that had to be overcome.** In this situation I was able to figure out how to safely use a variety of clamps and other holding devices that enabled me to do the job.

I was diagnosed as having Charcot-Marie-Tooth (CMT) disease (instead of polio) in 1959, by a Chicago neurologist, Dr. Robert Tentler. However, no one could give me an accurate prognosis. I was told that I would live a fairly normal life physically speaking. The one exception to the belief that I would live a normal lifespan was my life insurance agent who charged me sky-high rates.

The CMT diagnosis was reaffirmed by Dr. Bernard Patton at Baylor College of Medicine, Houston, Texas, via a nerve biopsy. The TYPE 1A was determined by Dr. James Killian, also at Baylor. Should you be interested in a brief description of CMT check it out in the Merck Manual Home Health Handbook.

In my version of CMT I cope with an extremely invasive case. On January 16, 1960, at the age of 23, I married a very special lady in a little country church in Minnesota. College courses were finally completed in 1961 and I went to work for the State of Illinois in 1962. My work location was in Chicago's downtown Loop. We lived in Evanston, a next-door suburb of Chicago, and I commuted to and from my job via

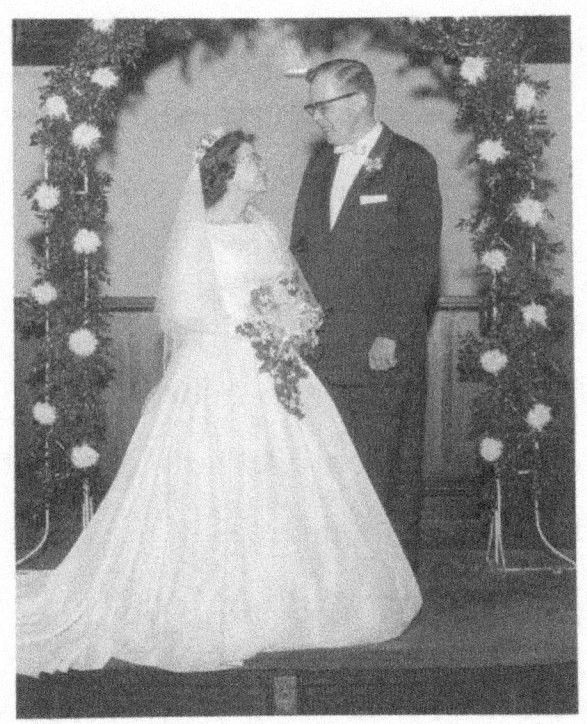

Our wedding on January 16, 1960

several trains. It usually took an hour to travel from my front door to my office door. In 1966 we received the gift of a son, Steven William, whom we adopted at age six weeks. We also had the privilege of taking into our little home for two years a young lady who was studying at the Spurtus College of Judaica in Chicago. Rita was a delight—a big sister for Steven—and another pal for Beem—our English Pointer rescued from the local animal shelter--who was with us for 9 years. We enjoyed tent camping together for 2 weeks in Wisconsin. Rita had a great work ethic and was the first Gentile to graduate from the Spurtus College of Judaica—she is fluent in Hebrew. Steven graduated from DePaul University, Chicago, with both BS and MS degrees in the computer field—and started his career with AMACO in Chicago.

During my 17-1/2 years of working in Chicago, I pushed myself and managed to carve out enough time to continue my education and earn a master's degree in Guidance & Counseling at Chicago's Roosevelt University which was about five blocks from my workplace. This meant four years of after-work-evening-school two evenings a week and included a Saturday practicum in my final year. My adviser, Dr. Abraham Simon, was demanding, tough and street-wise—having worked Chicago's streets as a MSW before earning his PhD. It was from him that I learned about the Neighborhood Settlement Movement that existed in the poverty pockets part of town. The time spent at Roosevelt was invaluable; at work it enabled me to make wise program development decisions. I received my MA degree in January 1970.

What made this all possible was that I was traveling around on my rebuilt right foot. In the mid 1960's a gifted surgeon rebuilt the foot via a triple-joint-fusion and movement of bone. At last the pain was gone and stability had arrived. However, due to on-going nerve damage and its resultant muscle loss,

my left foot was now a drop-foot and I wore a single bar steel leg brace to keep me from tripping.

Even though **my legs were growing weaker,** the changes were very subtle and I could manage traveling around town if I planned ahead where I was going—remember, this was before the ADA and curb cut outs. The trains were becoming more difficult to board. Also, I had to continue improvising different ways to **use my weak hands—even though a surgical attempt (in 1965) to preserve the strength in my left hand failed.** But it at least was a "try," and was done by a world renowned hand surgeon. Also note that my job with the State of Illinois required a lot of local travel both within the Chicago downtown loop or its surrounding area—and this in turn required greater use of my hands because of having to use them as wedges to haul my body up and down escalator and elevated train steps. But walking also took a growing effort due to the muscle loss in my legs. Fortunately, I had only one fall of note during my 17-1/2 years of working for the State of Illinois—I tripped on my brace falling flat on my face while crossing the lobby of the Pick-Congress hotel in downtown Chicago. Minimal help was offered for me to get up. I was an embarrassment to everyone present. Again, I had to bury my emotions.

My job duties with the State included program development, staff supervisor and trainer, employer relations, etc. I also traveled throughout the city and nearby suburbs. One of my notable accomplishments was developing a Manpower Training program for disadvantaged young men to learn the printing trade. I worked with the Printing Industry of Illinois Association at their training facility.

But my best memories belong to the last seven years of working for the State—I was the director of the Chicago Apprenticeship Information Center (AIC). My staff and I recruited gifted young people for formal apprenticeship opportunities in Chicago's building trade unions. I worked with the various building trades Apprenticeship Training Coordinators at their training facilities. Also, my staff and I promoted these opportunities via speaking at high schools and junior colleges throughout the city and nearby suburbs. We also administered, at our Center, a battery of aptitude tests to aid in the selection process. **I was too busy to think about the changes going on in my body.**

As I look back on these experiences, but for the grace of God, I don't know how I did it. Before entering an unfamiliar building, I had to "case" the place (especially if it was located in a poverty pocket part of town) for two reasons—to be sure that I could make a safe entry (no gang members hanging around) and that all handrails were in place because I could **not drag my legs up a step without a rail to hold onto**. I carried with me a catalog case and my briefcase—both crammed with promotional materials including two large reels of 16 mm film. I usually received needed help to carry the stuff once I got into a building—there was no smartphone invented as yet on which to call for help to get inside a building. Many times I would arrive in a good sweat. But, in spite of it all, I enjoyed the public speaking aspect of my job.

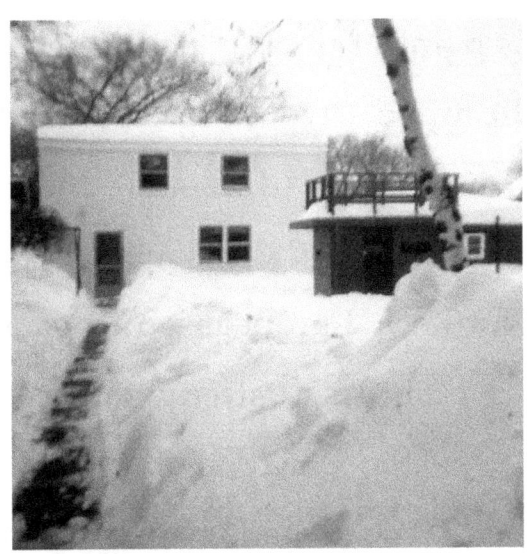

Blizzard "leftovers" – YUK!

Well, eventually the inevitable had to take place. Having survived one of Chicago's infamous blizzards the winter of January 1979, I had to face the fact that I could **no longer manage to travel on public transportation—my legs had continued to weaken and public transportation offered no assistance for people in my situation. I left my job in November 1979.**

At this point of my life, if you had told me that I was **handicapped** I would have denied it. I did not consider myself to be "different." I lived by the rule "where there is a will there is a way." Remember, the Swedes/Northern Europeans of my era were **stoic** and also **worshipped strength**. By choice I was oblivious to the fact that I was physically handicapped. (When handicap placards for vehicle use were introduced in Illinois it never entered my mind that I should apply for one.)

My Story

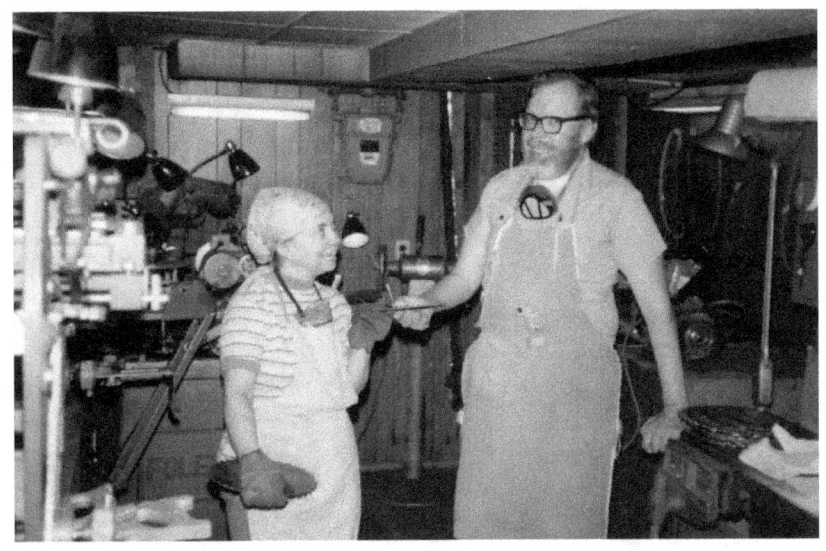

The machinists—my mate and I

What follows is an abbreviated version of the rest of my work life to date. In 1977, while I was still working in Chicago, we purchased a friend's business, including all necessary equipment; then by working part-time in the evenings, expanded a sharpening and tool grinding business serving the northern suburbs of Chicago.

The basement of our home now housed a machine shop. I did most of the shop work in the evenings and on Saturdays—my wife handling the surplus. We ran two routes per week. Initially, my wife and preschooler son picked up and delivered the goods serviced. But by the early 1980s I could no longer operate the business **due to the progressive weakening that I was experiencing in my hands and legs.** However, thanks to the business, the rear of our backyard was now occupied by a large 1-1/2 story building that was intended to house the machine shop but now offered space for both parking and a nice sized woodworking shop. Building it was a hands-on project and **I did my own contracting**. It took several years to complete. The building was well insulated, heated, and offered running water.

However, in spite of the growing weakening in my body, I could not leave well enough alone—we decided to **renovate a major portion of our house.** This turned out to be another several year project. Again, **I did my own contracting**.

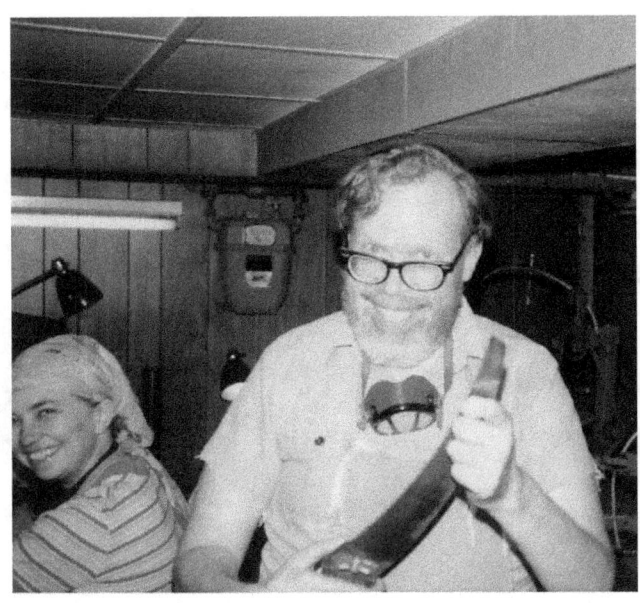

Yes, we're for real!

But thankfully, as this project neared completion, a major Change-Point appeared on the horizon—I met a clinical psychologist who directed me back into my field of academic training. He gave me training in his counseling techniques and referred some of his patients to me. His focus was on "Healing the Inner Child of the Past."

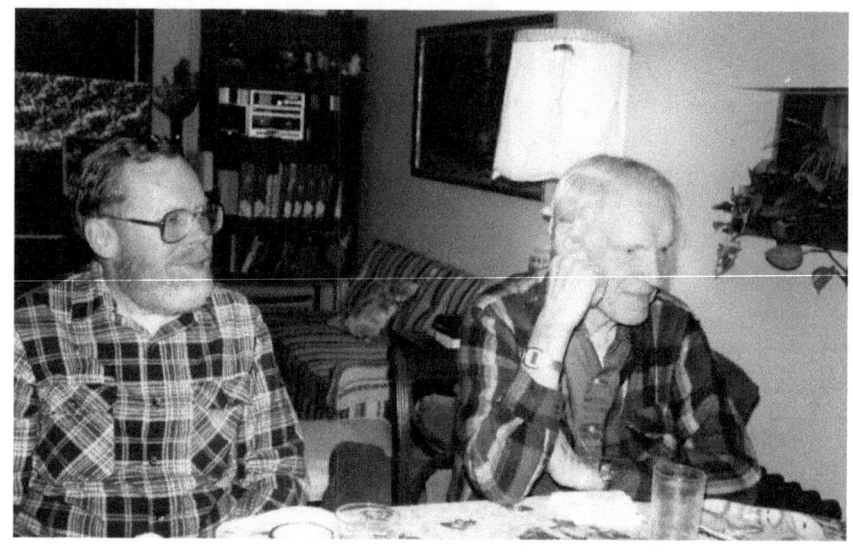

My mentor for 5 ½ years
Dr. James Stringham, MD
Birthday celebration time

Following a year spent with the psychologist, another training opportunity in the field of guidance and counseling developed. **I met a semi-retired medical-missionary-psychiatrist who gave me further counseling training and psycho-analysis. We met on a weekly basis for a period of 5+ years. James Stringham, MD, became the greatest mentor in my life.**

One of his areas of focus was the destructiveness that anger has on the human body. He held seminars on same at the annual meetings of the AMA and APA. His professional colleagues were just beginning to deal with this issue. Jim gave me written permission to use and disseminate his materials. Since both sets of our parents were deceased, my mate and I "adopted" Jim, a widower, as our father figure—what a privilege!

But now another problem surfaced—we could not escape the fact that the Chicago winters had gotten to us. We had barely survived another Chicago blizzard in January 1987. (But now I could **no longer hold a snow shovel** and I did not want my wife to be burdened with the shoveling chore. Also, her parents had a history of heart problems and strokes). **So in the fall of 1991 we made the big move to Houston, Texas.**

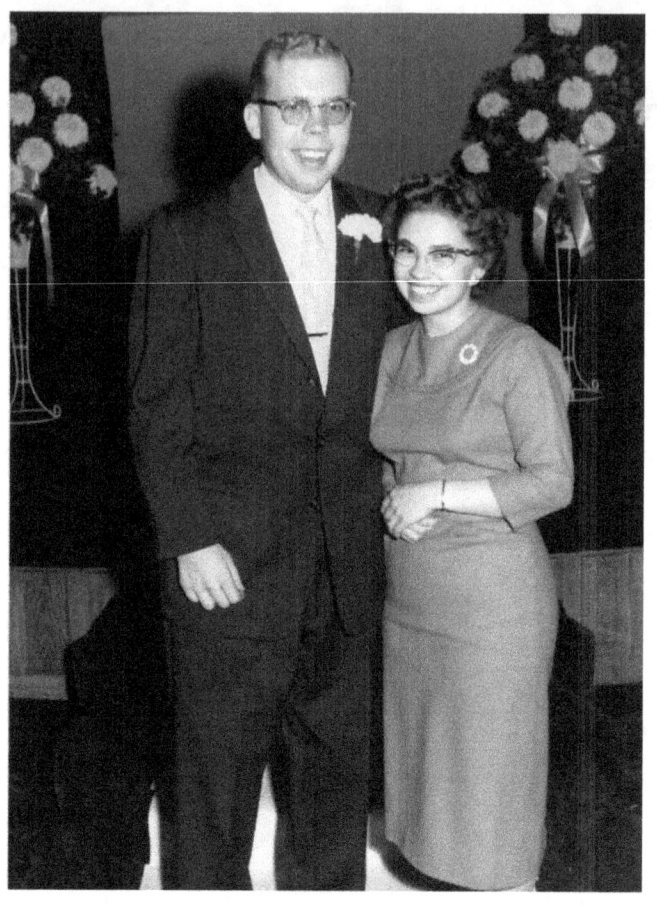

Another wedding anniversary to celebrate

But now another problem surfaced—we could not escape the fact that the Chicago winters had gotten to us. We had barely survived another Chicago blizzard in January 1987. (But now I could **no longer hold a snow shovel** and I did not want my wife to be burdened with the shoveling chore. Also, her parents had a history of heart problems and strokes). **So in the fall of 1991 we made the big move to Houston, Texas.**

Initially this proved to be a very difficult move. We only knew a few people. Back in Evanston our door was always open and we enjoyed helping each other out. Also, a small group of 15 people from our church met at our home on a weekly basis. But in Houston we didn't have such experiences. We felt isolated—dwelling behind tall wood fences and with neighbors who kept to themselves. It was like each man for himself. **Also, my medical and related resources were nonexistent and the disease was slowly progressing.**

Within five months my mate had a job as an executive secretary in the Texas Medical Center's Children's Nutrition Research Center (CNRC), working for three doctors (1M.D/1M.D.PhD/1PhD.)

who were engaged in the study of the nutritional needs of children.

I sat at home trying to do some writing and piddling around in our garage that we had converted into a very well equipped small commercial woodworking shop. It was our original intent when we moved to Houston to produce some small items such as high-end fancy boxes, etc. The building is well wired, insulated, has an A/C unit and a dust collection system. **But, as it has been the same story throughout my life, the neuromuscular disease dictated that such a dream would never come to fruition, i.e., I got weaker and the machinery was sold.**

I was not a happy camper—not licensed to practice counseling in the state of Texas and I did not have the physical strength to take the required additional academic courses demanded by the state. I could call myself a "consultant" but that did not open any doors nor generate any business. Neither am I a licensed Social Worker. I was on the threshold of having a nervous breakdown.

But finally an opportunity opened up to be a **full-time volunteer at The Institute for Rehabilitation and Research (TIRR)** also located in the Texas Medical Center. It was here that I **learned about assistive technology devices and products that would enable me to better function, physically speaking, in spite of the never ending weakening caused by the disease.** I was a full-time volunteer for five months, January through May of 1994.

Then, **in June of 1994, my wife heard of a job** opportunity that had opened up in the building where she was working—the Children's Nutrition Research Center (CNRC). I was hired as a staff member of the United States Department of Agriculture, Agricultural Research Service (USDA/ARS). This Agency built the facility and had a cooperative agreement with the Texas Children's Hospital (TCH), and Baylor College of Medicine (BCM)—in the operation of the building. The BCM staff of research scientists occupying most of the laboratory and related floor space—and, they were basically supported by generating their own grant monies. The USDA/ARS did maintain a small staff of their own research scientists—plus a three person office staff—I reported directly to the officer in charge.

Having been gone from the office environment for a number of years, I would have a lot of learning to do. It was a challenge and also forced me to make a major decision. **You see, I finally accepted the fact that I was physically disabled and had signed up for Social Security Disability. Accepting the new job meant that within a limited period of months I would no longer have the security of receiving a monthly disability check from the government. You** see, success in my new job would cause me to lose that valuable government check—I could not have both.

My decision was to take the job—which required the use of a computer—and I was basically computer illiterate. Also note that my body kept getting weaker. My new job duties included government bookkeeping, accounting, time-keeping, purchasing, supervisor of the building's office supply room, etc. The building was user-friendly with handicap rest rooms, easy access to elevators, the main doors, and underground parking for my altered van.

The job turned out to be a tremendous learning experience. My wife and I were even able to take a course in Medical Terminology at the Baylor College of Medicine.

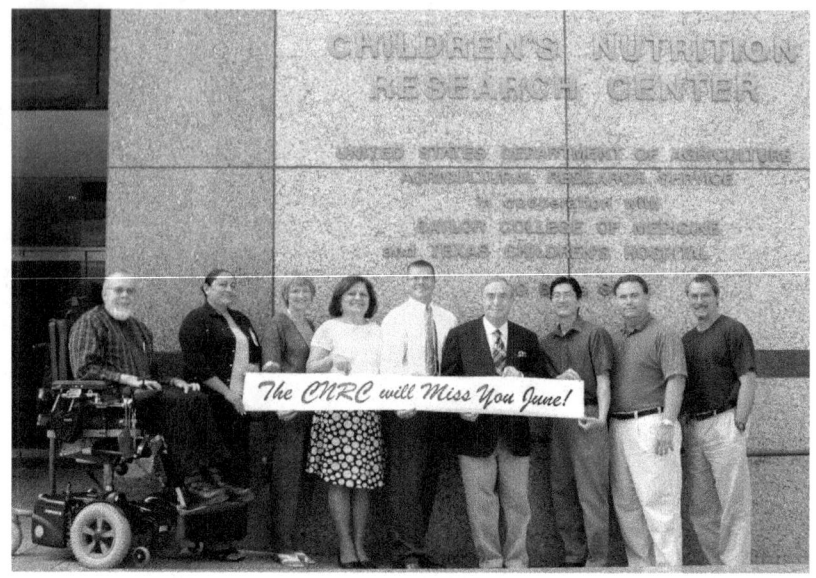

USDA-ARS staff with Dr. Bier, who was in charge of the CNRC Program

During the yearly **Disability Awareness Month** activities at work, I had the opportunity to organize the main event. The event was a grand gathering of the building's occupants for a good meal and a program that focused on the other side of the disability coin, namely "enablement." We enjoyed a variety of speakers, including Lex Frieden, who was one of the original authors of the ADA legislation.

I'll never forget the great time that we had when an organization brought their Service Dogs (with their trainers), who put on a very informative show for us. It's amazing the help that is available if you know where to look.

As you are well aware, sometimes good things come to an end. Such was the case of our respective jobs. **When we both turned 70 years old, and the weekly full-time work routine was taking its toll on our remaining strength—we decided to retire.**

By God's good grace we had been blessed in many ways. In 1995, we had purchased a large Ford van that was radically altered to accommodate my basic physical driving needs and also transported my power wheelchair and my wife's power scooter. The alterations enabled me to continue driving for a while. The State of Texas paid for all of the alterations. Also, prior to leaving our jobs, my health insurance agreed to pay for the purchase of a new power wheelchair—this was a much needed item.

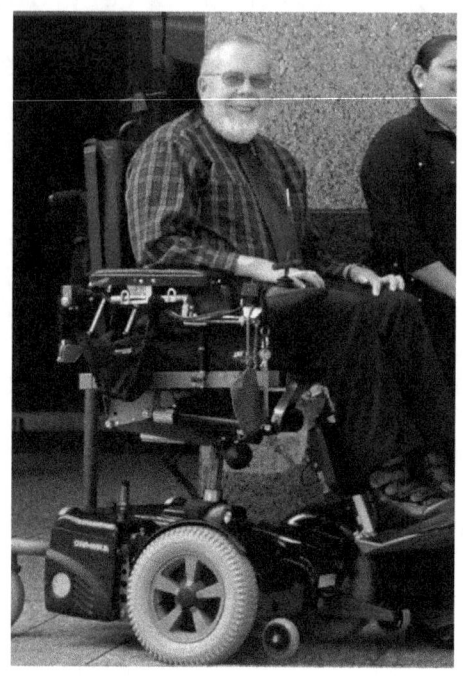

I wish you could see where I spent my working hours.
(see page 57)

Due to the insightful kindness of the USDA/ARS Administrative Officer on duty, Jimmy Goodman, I was equipped with a number of assistive products that enabled me to do the work assigned to me. Believe me, it was a joy to gather necessary information regarding these devices and other "helps." I discussed my needs with a gifted biomedical engineer, an occupational therapist, my physiatrist, neurologist, and the manager of the building's maintenance staff, etc.

Needless to say, I learned a lot in the process. If you are interested, check out the brief list at the end of this book to see what was for me **an accessible office equipped with assistive devices and other "helps." A maintenance mechanic at work who installed my assistive devices became a close friend and helper at home—John R. Osteen—a gift from God.**

Our official retirement date was the end of June 2006. However, we contracted our services at the CNRC and USDA until approximately mid-September 2006. Finally, it was time to slow down. In spite of life's trials and tribulations caused by the neuromuscular disease, with God's ever present help, we had experienced meaningful lives in the employment side of life.

So take heart, friend, I personally believe that God has plan and purpose for our lives. **"Trust in the Lord with all your heart, and lean not on your own understanding; In all your ways acknowledge Him, and He shall direct your paths." A quote from the book of Proverbs, Chapter 3, verses 5-6.**

But I must say that God's ways are sometimes difficult to understand and we have to hunker down and hold onto the way He wants to work out His plan and purpose for our lives on planet Earth. I also find sustaining strength in reading God's Holy Bible.

During our initial time at home we found daily enjoyment in being at home, building a few things in our woodworking shop (my mate now operating the machinery), enjoying our backyard flower beds, spending hours reading on the patio, etc.

But in November/December 2009, our lives changed a lot. It started with my fall in our bedroom (no broken bones), but it seemed to accelerate the progression of my neuromuscular disease. I became measurably weaker. I also developed a case of shingles in spite of having previously taken the shingles vaccine. Several weeks later, via an ambulance, I was taken and admitted to The Methodist Hospital, which is located in the Texas Medical Center. After gratefully enduring what seemed to be every test known to man, nobody could figure out why I lost most of my strength. Three and one half weeks later (which included 2-1/2 weeks in rehab) I was back at home.

Now we had to make major changes in our lifestyle. I no longer was able to bear weight on my

legs. So, I had to learn to use a transfer board—with assistance. I spend my nights in a motorized hospital bed. My 16 hour days are spent in my fully adjustable **power wheelchair.**

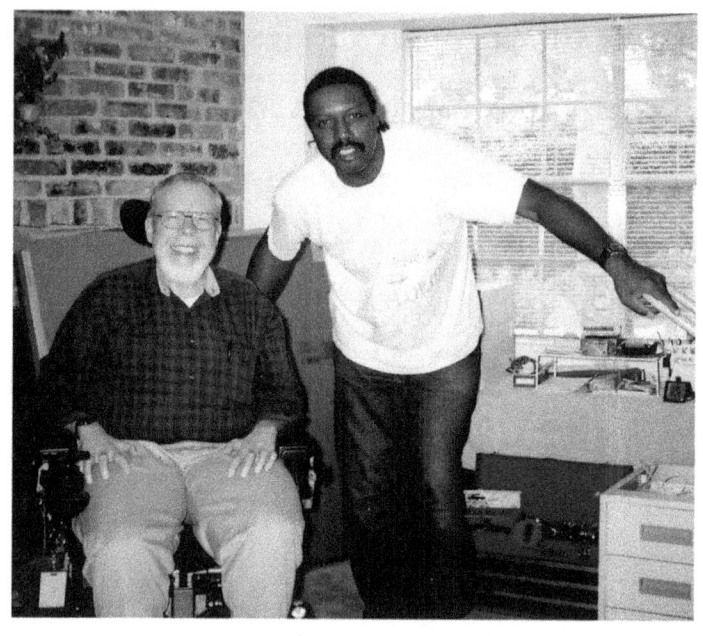

Myself and "Big John"—our special friend from work, John Osteen, who has the gift of helps

My faithful wife provided my **primary care** for the first 14 months that we were home from the hospital—a tremendous effort on her part. We then contracted with a home healthcare agency (CareWorks) for **caregivers** to stay with us from 7:00 p.m. to 7:00 a.m., seven nights a week.

However, our caregivers soon had two people to watch over. On January 2, 2011, my **wife experienced a heart attack** and it was then that we discovered my mate had some **serious cardiovascular problems** that we did not know about—some mini-strokes and artery blockages. But we are blest that, under the care of our gifted physicians and Jesus, our Messiah, she continues to exhibit remarkable recovery.

We also experienced another necessary financial blessing for both of us—we are now experienced enough to **screen our own caregivers. We have currently been blessed with very good caregivers.**

Now what about the future? Living is not over. We look forward to what the future holds for us— knowing that God holds our future in His hands.

Writing and working on our website will occupy a good-sized chunk of my time. My mate is getting **her interests** back on line—including lots of reading, handling the office work, some household chores, etc. In addition to the January 2nd heart attack, an MRI of her brain revealed a history of mini-strokes that were responsible for short-term memory loss. However, she has now experienced major recovery of ground lost in this most crucial area of daily living. We are grateful that God gives us necessary strength and provision for each day.

Another consideration: **as part of one's physical disability baggage there is a small package marked "disappointing experiences." Most of us would just as soon forget many of our "yesterdays."**

I've already shared with you a number of CMT related disappointments in my life. Another big one was the **loss of my baritone voice**—in spite of the fact that I had taken voice lessons while in college.

(After singing at a wedding I had even sparked the interest of a booking agent.) But in my early '20's my vocal chords started to "weaken" for no apparent reason. My father, who had an extremely mild case of CMT, had a similar experience, as did my sister—whose visible CMT on-set was much earlier in life than mine. However, there was a bright side in that enough of my voice remained to enable me to sing in a men's quartet for several years. Life was certainly not all gloom and doom!

I have now taken you through the abbreviated version of my story. This might not be your typical disability story, but you probably can identify with me at some point as you read my story. I have no doubt that I can identify with many of your stories, be you afflicted with a nerve or muscle based problem, and are a paraplegic or quadriplegic.

When I write I try to keep in mind the huge question, namely, **"how do we then cope in the**

multi-compartments of life when we have a physical disability?" Obviously, there are no easy answers. Don't think that I didn't seek good guidance throughout my life.

However, **the non-disabled world does not have a clue of what we live through day-by-day**. Nor can it understand the impact that physical disablement has on family and friends. Many people "disappear" from one's life if a disablement drags on-and-on. Even so, we still have much to be thankful for.

No matter the number of years I have tucked under my belt, to still be of service to the disabled community remains my desire **regardless of my physical state**. As already stated, I believe that our lives have God-given value and purpose, in spite of, and even because of, our physical limitations. We each have a story to tell and I look forward to disseminating pertinent information with you.

If some of you would like to share your story with me, please do so. Just let me know whether or not I can share your story with my audience. Note: Some physically disabled people struggle with the question **"would my life have been lived differently if good guidance had been given at crucial Change-Points?"** This question needs to be thought through very carefully before answering. Guard yourself from a root of bitterness. Down the road, I plan to discuss this question with you in our website.

I would appreciate receiving your comments about "My Story." As you can read between the lines, I believe when God's door of opportunity opens it needs to be investigated. If it is something that I think I am qualified for and can handle, I go-for-it!

Also, I never got hung up constantly looking for that "dream" career position. Please keep in mind that the ability to work is a privilege and there is nothing dishonorable about working in a menial "job" or a series of such "jobs." All legitimate work is of value. Remember that a "job" could lead you into a career. If, because of missed or nonexistent opportunities, you cannot learn to do what you like—why not learn to like and become productive in the opportunities that are available to you?

I now have given you a partial picture of my life. We've also engaged in other work related activities. Maybe we will have opportunity to share more with you at a later date—probably on our website. Thanks for reading.

John E. Tapper
sunburst@hal-pc.org

P.S. Currently I require the services of others to successfully travel thru a day. How grateful we are for each and every one of you.

During the month of December 2013, we spent another week at The Methodist Hospital. However, we do admit that it's **hard to be at the hospital when there is so much to do—so much to write about.**

John E. Tapper

My Story

ASSISTANCE FOR LIVING –
QUESTIONS

For Self Evaluation and Identifying New Options

Questions: Do you think surgery and/or adaptive equipment would enable you to live a more productive life? If so, what surgery? Or, what adaptive equipment?

Questions: Why do you suppose no adult (medical personnel, parents, or other adults, with the one exception of my grandmother) ever discussed my physical problems with me? [Some obvious answers include not knowing what to say to me, living with the wrong diagnosis of polio, etc.] Now, does any of this apply to you and your circumstances? If so, how does this affect you? What help do you need to better cope with your problem?

Questions: I had several reasons for attending college. These included escaping from the physically exhausting work experienced in the laundry, most of my friends were enrolled in college, and I felt the need to discover what I should do with my life. Are these valid reasons for attending college? Because my neuromuscular disease was progressive, what else should I have been addressing? Do you need to set new priorities?

Questions: Do you constantly have to prove yourself physically capable of performing in a variety of work place assignments? If so, what are you being asked to do that pushes your limits? How do you compensate for your nerve-muscle loss? Are those who evaluate you fair in their assessments?

Questions: From reading My Story, do you think I was living in a state of denial? What about you?

Questions: If my choices were driven by necessity—what about yours? Do you think I made the right choices? If not, what should I have done differently? Why? Is there anything you need to begin doing differently?

Questions: Were my physical activities initially okay for me to be involved in? Should I have investigated other options? Do you think you need to reassess your physical activities?

Questions: Do you think I was finally on the right track regarding my past training? Should I have regrets for many of the major decisions made over the years? How could I profit from them? Do you have regrets? If so, how can you profit from them, going forward?

Questions: Would you agree with me if I said that my last job was one of the wisest employment choices I have ever made? Have you made a wise career choice? What are your options? What do you think would be your most wise career choice in light of your health?

John E. Tapper

ASSISTANCE FOR LIVING
OTHER NOTES OF INTEREST

AQUATIC THERAPY:

Whenever we had the opportunity to involve ourselves in a physical activity that we hoped would not hasten our physical demise, we would try to involve ourselves in same. Such was the case for aquatic therapy. And, we worked with some excellent aquatic therapists.

Originally, we had to take off from work in the early afternoon, drive to the pool, put on our swimwear, run through our exercise routines, shower, change clothes, and return to work. We did this two times per week. However, we could not keep this up indefinitely. We couldn't justify taking so much time off from our work.

So we found another facility that allowed us to run through our aquatic exercises in the early morning hours. By early, this meant to get up at 3:30 a.m., pack our stuff, be at the pool at 5:00 a.m., and engage in aquatic therapy for one hour. My mate would also swim a number of laps. At 6:00 a.m., we had to shower, get dressed for work, grab a bit of breakfast and get to work by 7:30 a.m. We did this routine 2 to 3 times per week for 4+ years. This ended when the neuromuscular disease weakened my legs to the point that I could no longer safely slide into the pool from my power-chair, nor could my hands/arms help me back into my power-chair. So, in the Fall of 2004, with deep regrets, we could no longer engage in aquatic therapy. You see, the pool did not have a lift and the powers to be had no intention of purchasing one.

For my mate and me, aquatic therapy was worthwhile. But I doubt that many people could understand the amount of physical effort that it took to pull off this caper. Remember, I am power wheelchair dependent. My mate had to assist me in the shower and dressing departments. This was no mean feat. But once again -- it was worth the effort expended.

SERVICE OPPORTUNITIES:

Just because our bodies are wearing out, we can still make a meaningful contribution to mankind, drawing from a lifetime of training and relevant experiences—we share with you some examples of the same:

In the early 2000's, we served on an advisory committee in Austin, Texas, monitoring a grant program that was focused on a service to the mentally challenged—developing a "Plan for Achieving Self-Support" (PASS).

My mate gave me invaluable input and support. The physical effort involved driving our modified van to Austin, TX. Because we were not always able to find a user-friendly hotel that accommodated my disability, it was quite tiring, but well worth the effort.

In the early 2000's, we also took a certified training program—in the "Parent as Case Manager" for the mentally challenged. Again, my mate gave me invaluable input and support.

CONFRONTING PERSONAL STUFF:

In the late 1990's through early 2000's, my mate and I participated in a series of weekend seminars—a Bible-centered self-development program that challenged us to identify, confront and resolve problem areas in our lives that needed to experience personal growth.

None of these seminars were a walk in the park, as we made public and dealt with major issues in our lives that we needed to face, were held responsible for, and discovered workable solutions. We worked on a one-on-one basis together with a coach, then in a small group, and finally with the entire gathering. We appreciated the opportunity to attend. They were usually held on weekends. Through these seminars, we experienced a needed renewing of our minds.

John E. Tapper

My Story

ASSISTANCE FOR LIVING
Equipping the Office

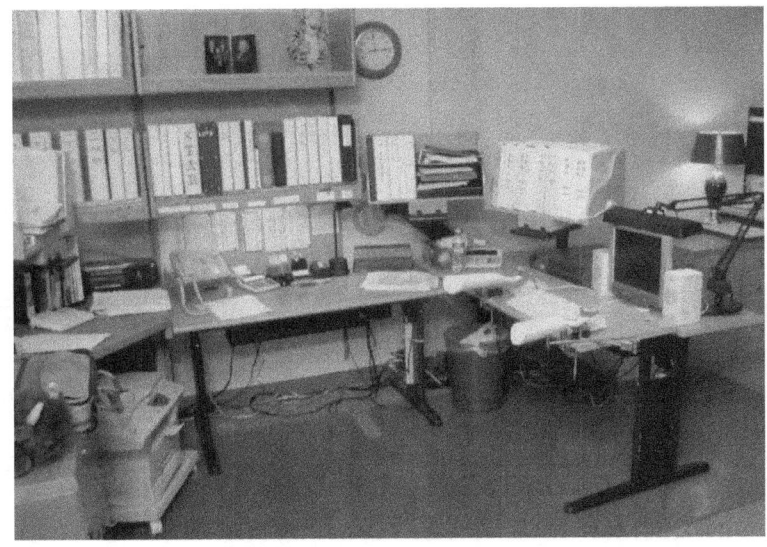

My office at work

The following is a list of assistive devices and adaptive equipment that enabled me to perform my job duties while working for the USDA: (Thank you to Administrative Officers' Jimmy Goodman for the purchasing approval, and Perry Rainosek for ongoing support.)

   *   A two piece, two motor driven (raise-lower) computer work station.

   *   A one piece motorized (raise-lower) work desk.

   *   Computer-use-assists designed and fabricated by the biomedical engineer. Basically, I hit the keyboard with rubber-tipped rods. The rods are attached to swiveling arm-troughs, which, in turn, are attached to a neat system of welded rods and swivel joints. The entire apparatus is attached to my computer workstation.

Some years back I had started computer use with elastic cuffs that held eraser-tipped pencils. Then, as my hands weakened, a friend fabricated for me a pair of portable metal devices that held those eraser-tipped pencils. When I could no longer handle these devices, my biomedical engineer came to the rescue. His devices are what I am now using as I work at the computer in my home office.

* Dragon Dictate software for writing text—limited use at work but heavy use at home.

* Three "floating" bookcases that were within my reach in which my three ring binders and other materials were housed. Basically put, these were finished rectangular wood boxes mounted on swiveling wall-mounted hardware designed to hold a TV set.

* A very high-end adjustable commercial desk chair that I could still transfer into. Cost- $3,000.00

* A commercial multi-function fax, copy, print, and scan machine—mounted on a rolling base that was within my reach.

*   Electric: three-ring punch, letter opener, stapler and adding machine—reduced effort to use.

*   File drawers accessible from my desk-chair—included was a large five drawer lateral file that had large leather made-to-order loop straps attached to each file door that I could slip my hand and wrist through to pull the drawers open. The letter file drawers had custom metal drawer pulls designed for my use.

*   A custom-cut polycarbonate floor mat provided zero resistance as I rolled in my desk chair.

Thoughts to Muse Over

WALLS

I build my little world inside the safety of my walls. There is no door for those that could befriend to pass through. Only the very daring would chance to climb over uninvited. But truth and heart knows the inner cry, the deep yearning that someone would at least try to penetrate and thus become a needed guest in the tiny chamber that I call life. Help me to break down my walls, so thick and crusty they've become. The scars of life have made them so, the load too heavy for me to bear.

Yes, walls were made to bring relief within the privacy of my soul. But shutting out means, shutting in, no freedom here if you must know. Won't someone care to stand alongside and help me chisel walls away? It will take time and lots of strength to stay with me for many a day. Is there a friend somewhere who cares to undertake a task so great?

To help set me free to face reality involves difficult choices for both you and me. But a deep inner yearning now captivates me--"Oh God, let me be what you've made me to be." A battle does wage on but freedom draws near—the walls of my life, no longer held dear.

John E. Tapper
AnAbleWord

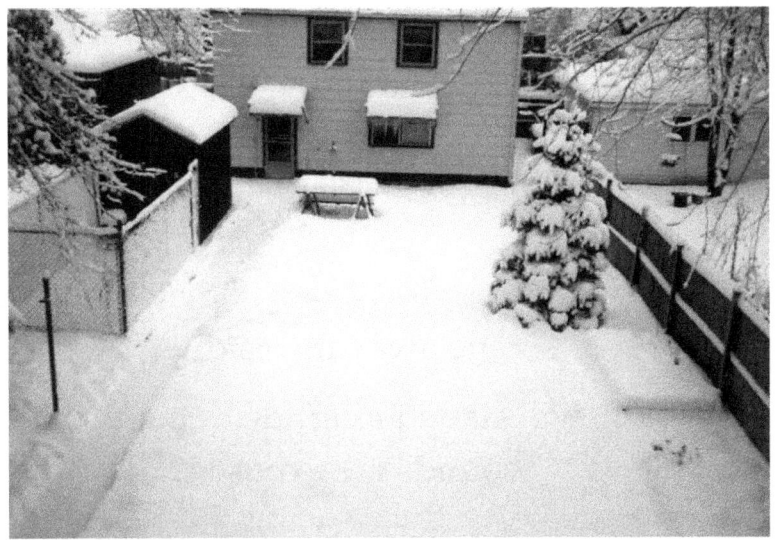

*The fruits of our labor resulted in what you see.
These included the dog run, garden shed, picnic area and
Large shop/garage. A view from our house.*

FROST

The frosts of many seasons lays heavily on my heart,

its grasping tentacles envelop my soul

and shut out the real world of feeling and response.

When, O Lord, will this long winter end?

When will the temporary cease and permanence be restored?

John E. Tapper

Where did my roots go? Have they died? Been cut off?'

Or are they resting, waiting to be fed, restored?

Who will help me? Who will melt the frost and scrape away its residue?

Who will stand alongside as many painful wounds are exposed?

I function differently now.

Can my soul be restored to walk this earth in happiness and peace?

Do I expect to be accepted as I am?

Melt all the protective frost, O Lord.

Use whatever means to help. I accept Your work within.

You hear my cries, my pleas.

A fresh start Lord-grant me this gift.

Though the past is always with me,

My Story

I choose to allow the melting of the frost,

its purposes now served.

Who exists beneath its many layers?

I must make decisions.

A fragile wholeness returns, a miracle, a work of Your grace!

Your Book speaks truth.

I am responsible.

Yes, free of frost,

free at last!

John E. Tapper
AnAbleWord

Food for Thought: Living in a temporary state on a permanent basis is extremely destructive! Forgiveness cannot take root until the "frost" has melted!

EVERYONE HAS A STORY

The couple I met at Wal-Mart had lost their son. They cared for him at home. He died from cancer years ago. He did not want to die in the hospital. The parents still bear and feel the pain, especially at the holidays.

So what did they do? They operated a small craft table at a local Wal-Mart selling their little craft items, the money going to Texas Children's Hospital in Houston.

Wow! Raising money while coping with a never-ending pain. Yet they smile through a pain that sprouts deep within their hearts of loss.

There are many stories like this and they all involve coping with, and accommodating, a pain of loss that resides deep within. Yes, dear reader, everyone has a story.

John E. Tapper
AnAbleWord

My Story

AN ELDER'S STATEMENT

My needs are basic, don't you see?
Yet shoved into a corner is not to be.
Honor bestowed is part of God's plan,
So much to share, listen if you can.

My eyes still contain a sparkling glint,
but the years have left their indelible print.
A change in color as gray turns the hair,
Mapping the skin, wrinkles are there.

If a place to call home is part of God's plan,
Familiarity, so important, tells who I am.
Regardless how modest surroundings may be,
A comfort so priceless it offers to me.

Of trials, no stranger to this elder they are,
The wheel of the Potter shaping clay from afar.
The Son's image, so precious, emerging you see,

And the shaping will continue to eternity.

Now patiently awaiting the summons from above,
A desire to be useful is bathed in God's love.
Come now then and learn from "elder wisdom" freely given,
A "surround of blessing" will be yours from Heaven.

John E. Tapper
AnAbleWord

Food for Thought: A focus on self-preservation is not to be--then life gets centered around the big "I." The "look out for number one" syndrome can easily reestablish itself-so watch out!

My Story

A NEW NORMAL

Deeply moved by words that represented
a world that was so different.
Oh why did such radical change
have to take place deep within my being?

"Newness" was always something sought for,
but "mistakes" negated any gains made."
A "new normal" is what "they" say I need
as I live day by day.

But from a physical point of view
my new normal is not static--
my body constantly changing.
The slippery slope of "accommodation"
has become
my new normal.

John E. Tapper
AnAbleWord

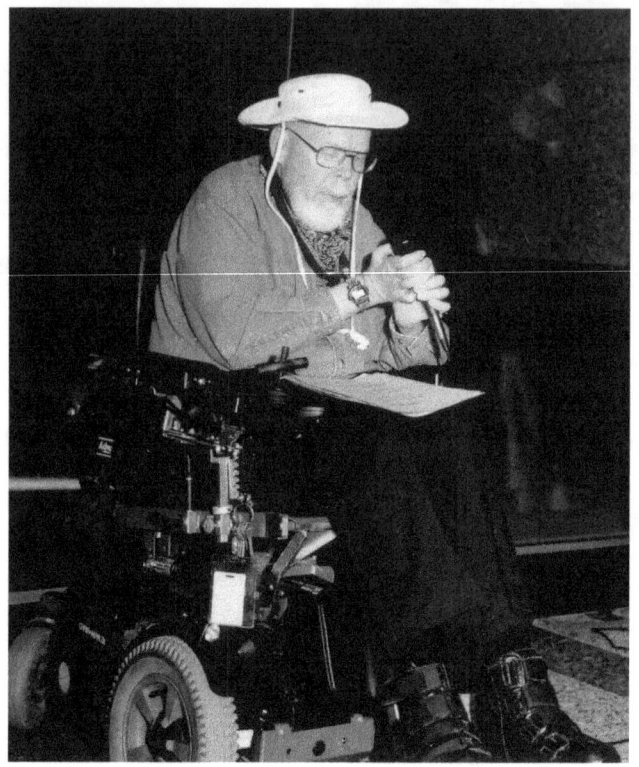

*Sitting in my wheelchair,
the music of yesteryear, playing in my memories.*

Food for Thought: "New Normals" are not necessarily of profit, especially if they embrace the negatives of life.

My Story

PEELING PAINT

Peeling paint brings back memories of a time so long ago.
The old homestead, now vacant, is basking in the sun's warm glow.
The laughter of yesteryear's children still echoes in the rooms and the halls.
Their joy being so contagious as they play with their old rubber balls.

I wonder about the many stories told by generations past.
The joys, and the storms of a lifetime, that were weathered by those who held fast.
Their faith, so strong and non-moving, withstood the many tests of time.
I think that I now understand it, the hard work, the sweat and the grime.

I remember the winds, storms and drought that drove so many to leave.
But my people turned to their God who sustained them while they did grieve.
Yes, with tears in my eyes I now see that memories remain to be freed
by an old building standing before me, peeling paint, and still meeting my need.

    John E. Tapper
    AnAbleWord

John E. Tapper

My Story

NIGHT

The moon gently splashing it's light on the waters,
Tall pines are revealed in the forest nearby.
The call of the loon pierces the semi-silence.
Insects waking up, noisy, their presence known.
The water's gentle rippling makes friends with the shore.

Sand castles of yesterday, disappearing, are no more.
An old boat rocking as in a cradle, creaking, groaning.
Oars bereft of paint, edges worn, rough, are waiting.
Cabin light escapes thru unwashed window panes.

Firewood, neatly stacked, makes its needed contribution.
Wisps of smoke curl from chimney, adding fragrance.
The movement of a rocking chair, noise so familiar.

John E. Tapper

Precious moments of the past, can they not return?

City night descends upon us with its noisy wake-up calls.
Windows barred from intruders gives assurance to us all.
Sirens scream their right-of-way as we journey to the mall.

Overcome by the flow of new knowledge, mankind explodes!
Growing wiser day-by-day is what the "experts" seem to say.
New understandings we may have, but what about the night?
Erasing darkness is the goal, streetlights shining everywhere.

Urban dwellings, why hold on to see them self-destruct?
The price of greed, collapsing buildings, codes to build ignored.
Air polluted, lungs turn black, we cough and wheeze in despair.

My Story

Finally screaming out in need, Not fair! Not fair! Not fair!

Precious moments of the past, can they not return?
Is darkness to take over and envelop us with fear?
Night should be a precious time, freed from toil, and snare.
A time to rest and be refreshed, held tightly in God's care.

Those precious moments from the past, they do now return.
The gift of memory, freely given, reflects upon the yesteryears.
So, freed from fears of city life, memories bring peace and joy,
The simple life that once was lived, in memory will not die.

John E. Tapper
AnAbleWord

John E. Tapper

My Story

"TRUGGELING"
(Traveling Thru Struggles)

Our road is one of being trod as hand in hand we tightly clasp.
"Children" looking for some answers,
"Elders" wondering where to find them.
Why the struggle to exist? Why the battle long we've fought?
Where is the answer bright and clear, to tide us over and give new song?

The years pass by like fleeting clouds.
The yesterdays rolled up as one. Visions dimmed by promises broken,
The soul pierced deep by "tokenism."
So we trod the path of life, wanting still to see the change.

How long, O God, we sit and wait to hear a vibrant fresh new song?
And yet we "truggel" still hand-in-hand,
Daring, believing, that life will change.
Looking for new hope tomorrow,
Answers that will mend our souls.

John E. Tapper

Facing the door of deep desire,
Turning the key in the rusty old lock.
Destroying the thoughts of "toleration,"
Freedom to "truggel" is not for naught.

Our struggling subsides, answers revealed,
Souls at rest, new hope to live by.
Choosing to walk in the "new life" freely given,
A gift from our Savior who lives on High.

John E. Tapper
AnAbleWord

My Story

If you would like to contact me,
please send an email to:

John E. Tapper
sunburst@hal-pc.org

A website has been created
to help fund my medical care.
If you are
interested please go to:

gofundme.com/gvj87c

Sunburst Services
2014

Front Cover Design and layout by
MOZ ART & Co.

John E. Tapper

My Story

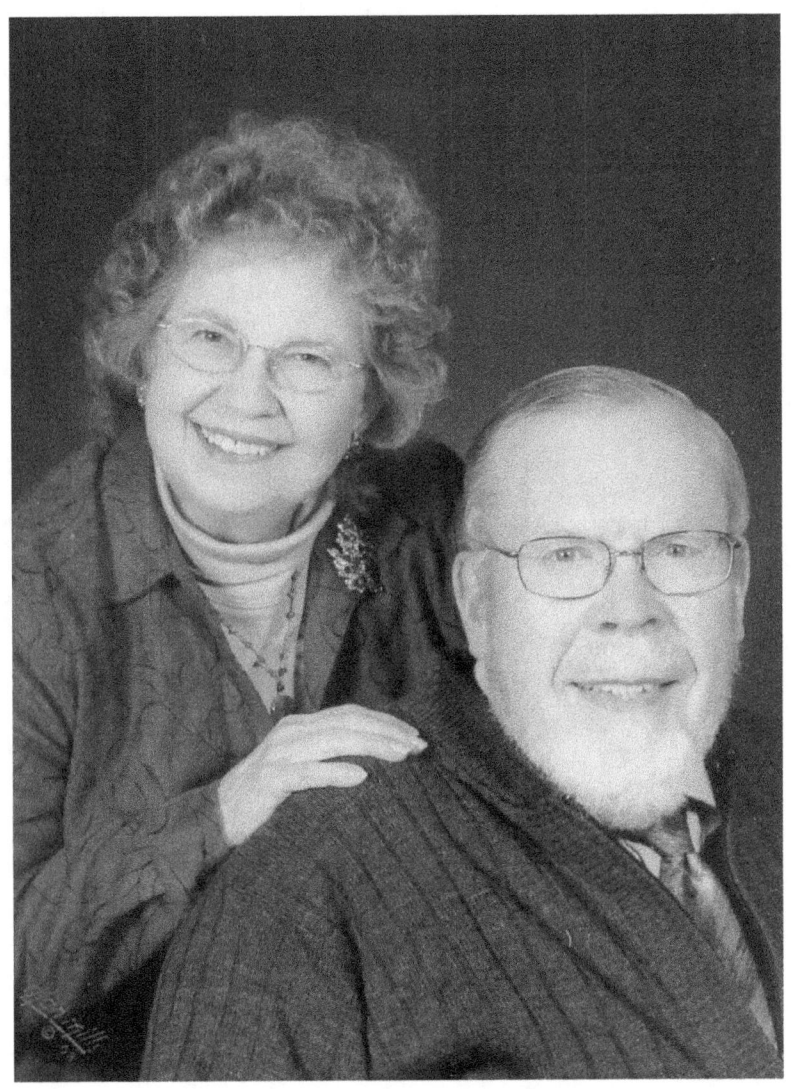

John and Idelle Tapper

www.ingramcontent.com/pod-product-compliance
Lightning Source LLC
Chambersburg PA
CBHW071749170526
45167CB00003B/988